Gluten Free Bible: A Complete Guide to Living Gluten Free

What You Need To Beat Celiac Disease with the Gluten Free Diet

By: Debbie Blaine

9781632874597

I0413970

PUBLISHERS NOTES

Disclaimer – Speedy Publishing, LLC

This publication is intended to provide helpful and informative material. It is not intended to diagnose, treat, cure, or prevent any health problem or condition, nor is intended to replace the advice of a physician. No action should be taken solely on the contents of this book. Always consult your physician or qualified health-care professional on any matters regarding your health and before adopting any suggestions in this book or drawing inferences from it.

The author and publisher specifically disclaim all responsibility for any liability, loss or risk, personal or otherwise, which is incurred as a consequence, directly or indirectly, from the use or application of any contents of this book.

Any and all product names referenced within this book are the trademarks of their respective owners. None of these owners have sponsored, authorized, endorsed, or approved this book.

Always read all information provided by the manufacturers' product labels before using their products. The author and publisher are not responsible for claims made by manufacturers.

This book was originally printed before 2014. This is an adapted reprint by Speedy Publishing, LLC with newly updated content designed to help readers with much more accurate and timely information and data.

Speedy Publishing, LLC

40 E Main Street,

Newark

Delaware

19711

Contact Us: 1-888-248-4521

Website: http://www.speedypublishing.com

REPRINTED Paperback Edition: ISBN: 9781632874597

Manufactured in the United States of America

DEDICATION

This book is dedicated to all those who fight to have more gluten free products available where they live. My aunt had to travel lots of mile to get her food.

When you have a disease that restricts what you can eat you start to value the availability of things that much more.

TABLE OF CONTENTS

Chapter 1- Gluten-free: A Smart Choice or a New Trend

Not long ago, the term "gluten-free" was thought to only be for those who suffered serious health issues in regard to gluten intolerances. Today, however, many individuals are choosing to live a gluten-free life.

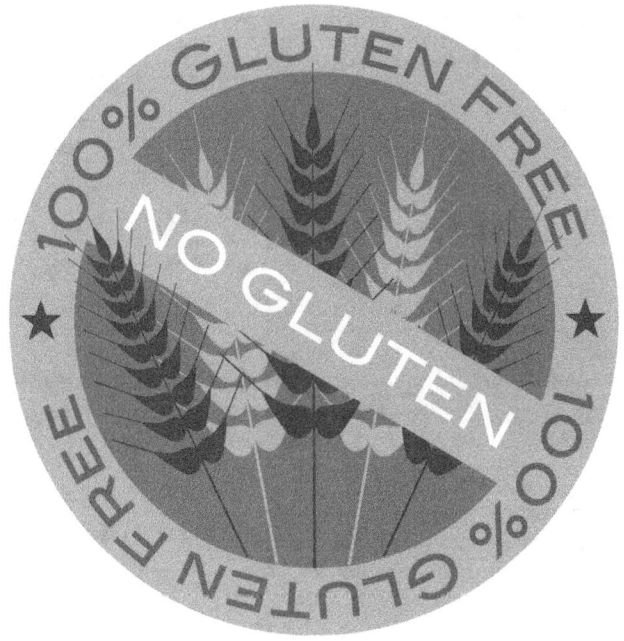

There are many reasons people will opt for a gluten-free diet. Some are more obvious than others and include:

- Celiac disease
- Gluten intolerance
- Wheat allergies

- Inflammatory processes
- Personal choice

Celiac Disease

When particles of gluten bond with intestinal proteins and generate a hypersensitive overreaction from white blood cells, celiac disease can develop. The small intestine plays an integral role in this process as they are designed to absorb nutrients. With Celiac Disease, however, the small intestines cannot do their job properly because the body's white blood cells incorrectly identify the gluten bond particles as an enemy and therefore set out to destroy the lining of the small intestine.

Some of the symptoms of celiac disease are associated with other diseases though so blood tests are typically necessary to properly diagnose the problem. Some of those symptoms you may experience with Celiac Disease are as follows:

- Abdominal pain
- Persistent diarrhea
- Bloating
- Constipation
- Vomiting
- Fatigue
- Weight loss

Gluten Intolerance

Word of mouth is a very powerful tool. Many individuals have opted to adopt a gluten- free lifestyle because someone that they know has touted the benefits from doing so. For most individuals, there are no real cut and dry answers as to whether he or she may have intolerance to gluten. Blood work along with an endoscopic biopsy of the small intestine will determine if the patient has celiac disease, however, there is not much in the way scientifically to report whether a person has gluten intolerance.

Many individuals claim to simply feel better when not eating products that contain gluten. These people state that living a gluten-free lifestyle simply leaves them feeling more energized, less bloated, and with clearer thinking capacities.

Wheat Allergies

Wheat allergies, however, are another story. An allergy, unlike intolerance, caused by gluten is a serious subject. When an antibody to wheat is produced, also known as an IgE, many allergic reactions will occur:

- Hives
- Redness
- Swelling
- Itchy eyes, nose, throat
- Cramping
- Vomiting and diarrhea
- And in worse case scenarios, anaphylaxis

Anaphylaxis can cause many serious side effects such as:

- trouble swallowing
- difficulty breathing
- chest pain
- tightening of the throat
- an accelerated heart beat Thankfully, these are the extreme cases.

Inflammatory Process

While there is no concrete evidence either medically or scientifically that going gluten- free is necessary for inflammation to decrease, many individuals who stick to a gluten- free diet believe that it does help.

Some individuals tout the benefits of being gluten-free as having more energy and feeling less bloated; but research does not support this as of yet.

Personal Choice

For those with true celiac disease, it must be hard to comprehend why anyone who did not have to would go on a gluten-free diet. Gluten-free products are extremely costly and definitely do taste differently.

Having said that, individuals become gluten-free for many reasons:

1. According to celebrities in the media, it is all the rage right now. Some individuals want to be trendy and follow those trends regardless of the reasoning.
2. Other consumers of gluten-free products say that they feel differently when eating a strictly gluten-free diet. Benefits such as more energy, less bloating, better memory are just a few of the claims made by individuals for going gluten-free.
3. Losing weight is a big motivator. Some individuals have pronounced the most positive effect of going gluten-free is the ability to lose weight and keep it off.
4. Avoiding things such as gas, bloating, cramping, and fatigue are a big bonus, as well.
5. Gaining more mental clarity is something that most everyone both male and female would appreciate obtaining.

Debbie Blaine

For many consumers, eating a diet without gluten simply makes them feel better, whether or not they are reaping any scientifically proven benefits and rewards

To avoid feeling the dreaded bloating often associated with eating gluten-filled foods, people may choose to go gluten-free. Bloat is something everyone experiences, some more than others. Women tend to get hit doubly during their menstrual cycle. So if there is even a slim chance to alleviate some of the gluten related bloating, many will be happy to give a gluten-free diet a try.

CHAPTER 2- WHAT ARE THE ADVANTAGES & DISADVANTAGES OF THE GLUTEN FREE DIET?

If you are a celiac sufferer, the benefits of going gluten-free are obvious. You get to alleviate some serious side effects to gluten including saving the lining of your small intestine from being under constant attack. Gas, bloating, vomiting, or diarrhea is side effects of gluten intolerance, as well.

If you are not a celiac sufferer, but instead are seeking the benefits of going gluten-free for the simple reason that it is the talk of town, you can still find many benefits from this change in diet. They include, but are not limited to:

1. Mental clarity may be a benefit. After removing gluten from their diets, many individuals report having more mental clarity. These individuals say that after months or years of "being in a fog" that the fog dissipates for them after being on a gluten-free diet. They also suggest that their memory loss and forgetfulness seem improves.
2. Fatigue seems to decrease. Consumers of a gluten-
3. free diet may find that his or her issues with sleep will improve once they remove gluten from their dietary intake. A better night's sleep and feeling less drowsy during the day may be good enough reasons for the sleep deprived to give the gluten-free lifestyle a try.
4. Maintaining weight is a desired goal. Losing weight and maintaining the weight loss is a desired goal for millions of people. Many people report that they were finally able to lose weight and keep it off after they changed their diet to be gluten-free.

5. Gluten could be life threatening. While mental clarity, fatigue and weight loss are all good reasons to give this diet a try, if you have celiac disease, going gluten-free can save your life.

For celiac suffers, even a tiny amount may have an adverse effect on the body. It can cause iron deficiency and anemia as well as Osteoporosis. Gluten can also set off a very serious reaction for some folks, including anaphylactic shock which can be fatal.

While many other individuals praise the fact that they are on gluten-free diets and tout benefits such as an overall feeling of well-being, energy increase, and alertness, none of these attributes have been conclusive in persons with only a small sensitivity to gluten.

For all of the good that a gluten-free diet does, it isn't without its faults.

The Disadvantages of a Gluten-free Lifestyle

Whole grains and wheat products have been a staple for the human diet for ages, and with good reason. By opting for a gluten-free lifestyle you might be unnecessarily eliminating vital nutrients your body needs to stay healthy. Four such nutrients include:

Niacin – Niacin helps to keep your skin, hair and eyes healthy. It assists with maintaining a healthy nervous and digestive system.

Niacin also helps convert carbohydrate into energy which is important if part of your goal for a gluten-free diet is to lose weight.

Iron - Iron has so many important jobs in our body. It carries oxygen to cells and carbon dioxide from them. It helps produce energy and hormones. Iron even plays a role in fighting against infections.

Vitamin B – Vitamin B has many parts and each part provides its own set of benefits. Generally speaking vitamin B is instrumental in maintaining a healthy immune & nervous system.

Zinc – Zinc may not be something you think about often, but its job is as important as any other nutrient. Zinc assists our immune system with responding to threats. It also plays a role in brain function and reproduction.

If you choose to seek out a gluten-free diet, you should consult with your primary care doctor before taking on this new lifestyle. In addition, you should be prepared to take a daily supplement to make up for any lost nutrients.

Nutrients may not be the only thing lacking in a gluten-free diet. Many people complain about the lack of variety available and taste in gluten-free foods. Gluten-free products definitely have a distinct taste and once you have eaten a certain variety of pasta for several years, you may never get used to the gluten-free kind.

Cost is another downside to this diet. Gluten-free products are very costly. Although you may be able to find gluten-free products on the shelves of supermarkets, they will still typically be expensive, especially while gluten-free continues to be the 'in fad' in the eyes of consumers.

Be prepared to become a label reading guru if you choose to go gluten-free. Gluten is found in many unsuspecting foods such as spaghetti sauce, soy sauce, and in some packaged products, as well. You will need to extremely wary of labels and plan to spend extra time shopping, at least in the beginning stages, if you are going totally gluten-free.

Debbie Blaine

Cooking at home is less expensive than purchasing prepared products; however, this can be time consuming and cumbersome. You can certainly buy gluten-free pancake mixes, muffin mixes, cake mixes, and bread mixes, but be prepared for a little bit of mess and some extra time involved in preparing your own gluten-free menus, especially if you start from scratch.

Dining out, eating at another person's home and vacationing can all be extremely difficult while trying to maintain the gluten-free lifestyle. You will need to make certain that your wait staff, hotel staff, and hosts are all aware of your lifestyle choices. If they won't indulge you, you may have to skip the event or prepare your own meal ahead of time and take it with you.

CHAPTER 3- HOW TO PREPARE GLUTEN-FREE MEALS

You do not necessarily have to shop in a specialty store that only sells gluten-free products. Many gluten-free foods today can be found in supermarket aisles and the frozen section of many health food stores. Items such as pancake mix, muffin mix, bread mix, cereals, desserts, snacks and even frozen breakfast, lunch and dinner meals can easily be picked up at most supermarkets and health stores.

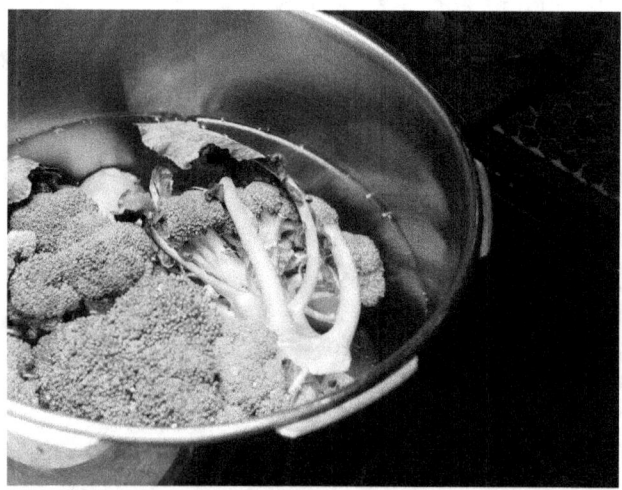

If you're planning on traveling for an extended time, be sure to visit the gluten-free section of your local supermarket and stock up on snacks. This will ensure you are prepared any delays at the airport, in traffic or in the event that where you are traveling to does not have a gluten-free section within the local stores. If you are headed out for a day trip, consider packing a lunch in a cooler so you can have a ready-made meal when you want.

Debbie Blaine

Preparing gluten-free meals really starts with understanding your grains and starches. You should read up on which grains and starches you can and cannot have as well as what you can use as a substitute. While you're reading, make a list of items you want to look for during your next shopping trip. Keep this list handy so you can take it with you and make notes if you find a brand you particularly like.

Always try small packages of mixes before buying a larger portion. You will find that some gluten-free flours make great muffins but not so great pancakes. Others might do well with biscuits but fall flat with a cake. So test out several to find which brands you like best for each food you make.

If you are planning to be 100% gluten-free, you should be aware of cross-contamination. Always store your gluten-free products separate from everything else. Before using any utensil, make sure it is free of gluten residue. If you can afford it, purchase a new toaster and other appliances that you can use strictly for your gluten meals.

Preparing your own gluten-free products from scratch is similar to batch cooking as you would with normal meals. You can prepare gluten-free pancakes and freeze the batter in separate, smaller containers for the future. Baking breads and muffins in batch form is also a great idea for your workweek. In addition, then there is always the option of preparing gluten-free wraps and filling them with ham and eggs or potatoes and vegetables for a yummy quick breakfast or lunch.

Another awesome idea is to make a gluten-free quiche for dinner and combine it with a salad. This will fill you up, give you vital vegetables such as broccoli and spinach, and keep you gluten-free and satisfied. Many individuals find that freezing individual slices of quiche make for a great breakfast starter or even lunch.

Be prepared. It is very important to be prepared when undertaking gluten-free baking. It is an art that needs to be learned and learned by the old adage of if you do not succeed at first, try, try, and then try again.

Be patient. Baking gluten-free takes some time and some practice. More than likely your first experience with gluten-free baking will not result in something that is just waiting to be photographed and placed in a magazine. It is a trial and error type of endeavor.

Reap the rewards. Once you have begun the process of trying gluten-free baking, you will notice that you will learn many nuances of gluten-free baking. You will find what works for you, in what amount, and how many ingredients. Stick with it and you will be pleasantly surprised that it will not only taste good to bake gluten-free, but it will feel good, as well.

You can use several different flour bases for your gluten-free baking:

- White rice flour
- Brown rice flour
- Coconut flour
- Almond flour

While the white rice and brown rice flour are a bit more traditional, the coconut and almond flours will add more sweetness and flavor to your base recipe.

Sweet rice flour may have a more starch-oriented base and can add a bit more moisture to your baking.

Buckwheat or quinoa flour will have a thicker and heavier component for your baking base.

As far as starches are concerned, potato starch and cornstarch are good choices for gluten-free baking.

If you are new to gluten-free baking, you will probably have to get used to baking with the additive known as xanthan gum. This is an added ingredient which will increase the thickness of your baking and have it stick together better. You will note as you first set out that baking gluten-free has the tendency to make your wares fall apart. The addition of xanthan gum, used sparingly, seems to alleviate this problem.

The nice thing, however, about gluten-free baking is that you can whip up a big batch of flour and dry ingredients and store it for later use. Adding things like yogurt, nuts (of course if no one is allergic), bananas, and raisins will all make for delicious tasty baked gluten-free goods.

CHAPTER 4- THE LINK BETWEEN GLUTEN AND AUTISM

It is important for every person to be health conscious and be more aware of the things that we do to our body especially to the food that we eat. It is important to know that the "good" foods presented to you are not always what they seem. Take gluten for example. Many people may not know the connection between gluten, autism and behavioral disorders like ADHD (Attention Deficit Hyperactivity), which can have negative effects on a person's personality like depression.

You may be surprised to know that gluten also is present to most of the processed food that we eat. Gluten can be very dangerous to everybody's health when eating it is not controlled.

Believe it or not it has also been proven to affect a person's behavior especially to those people who are already suffering from a disease particularly Autism and other behavioral disorders like ADHD (Attention Deficit Hyperactivity).

It has been known to be the source of neurological and psychiatric disorders for people who are sensitive to this protein.

For people with autism, taking in gluten can cause undesirable effects on their behavior. One major effect is that they suddenly become high which includes repetition in body movements as well as staring at particular parts of an object.

In other words gluten acts like opium for their body. That's why studies have shown that patients with behavior disorder show major improvements when on a gluten-free diet. Other diseases like bipolar disorders and schizophrenia which includes emotional breakdowns and delusions are also improved by excluding gluten from their diet.

Gluten as mentioned earlier is present in almost every food that we eat. That being said, if you happen to be one of those people who are recommended by your doctor to be on a strict gluten-free diet, you might find it very difficult to follow.

But you do not need to worry; nowadays various foods now come in a gluten-free variety. People who are intolerant with gluten need to follow a gluten-free diet to improve the health of the body and most especially the health of the mind.

We are haunted by the common misconception that wheat products are good and healthy for our body like what the food industry tells the people. It is very important to know that our body has the tendency to accept and also reject the food that we eat; oftentimes for most people their body finds gluten as foreign. As a result this may cause the body to attack some of your tissues even the good ones.

Gluten intolerance used to be rare among people, but with what's happening to our industry today, gluten sensitivity got spread among many people. You might not know that the reason behind a simple headache or a muscle pain is gluten and other wheat related food that you so enjoy eating every single day.

CHAPTER 5- HOW TO DETERMINE IF THE GLUTEN–FREE LIFESTYLE IS FOR YOU

Taking foods that are gluten free entails more than a change in diet. This is because one's lifestyle has to completely change, for instance, careful consideration of food has to be taken even when one is hungry but not act on impulse. The question that may run through your mind is: Is it worth adopting a gluten free lifestyle?

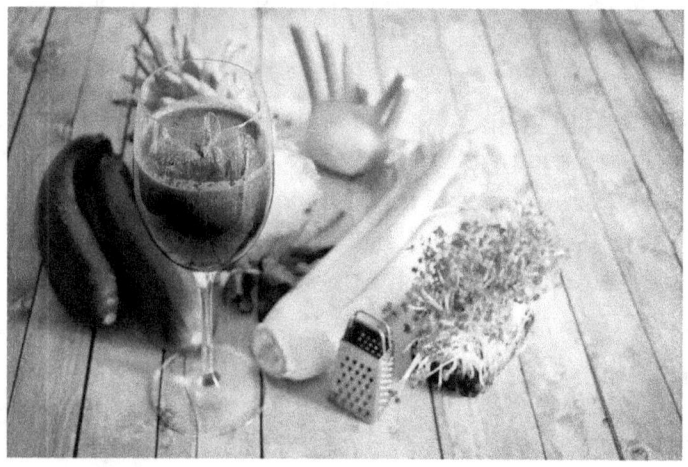

Reasons why people take to this kind of lifestyle:

There are three major reasons why people are opting to cut wheat and other gluten containing grains from their diet. These are:

1. Celiac disease - This is an inherited, autoimmune disease. Intake of more gluten leads to deteriorating the health of the patient as thier bodies are not able to digest this kind of protein. Grains containing this type of protein should therefore be eliminated from their diet.
2. Gluten intolerance - This is whereby the body produces allergic reactions and stomach cramps due to intake of

wheat or cereals containing gluten. This condition forces one to eliminate gluten in his or her own diet.

3. Healthy living - People have come to realize the importance of living healthy. Our bodies should be taken care of through the diet we take since our bodies are not designed to intake all kinds of food. Proper diet leads to weight loss in a healthy way and also eliminating possibilities of suffering from diseases like migranes, fatigue and depression.

Will your social life be affected?

Many people are worried about their social lives and places at which they can take meals when they adopt the gluten free lifestyle. Acquiring a gluten free lifestyle does not restrict you from attending social places or eating at restaurants. One can attend parties and social functions and still be careful on the choice of food you take. You can contact your host in advance to inform him or her on your condition.

There is a significant number of restaurants that offer special menus for gluten free foods. This is due to the increased number of people who are watching their diet. Therefore one does not have to make his or her own dish at home but can occasionaly eat out.

Before we cover it in a bit more detail in the next chapter, here are some of the benefits of living a gluten free life:

Getting rid of gluten in your diet and products that you use comes along with various and beneficial results. Some of these benefits are:

i. Reduced or eliminated chances of acquiring certain diseases such as cancer and diabetes.

    ii.   Weight loss - This type of diet does not contribute to gaining weight but can lead to weight loss.

    iii.   The diet helps people suffering from autism spectrum disorder - This is scientifically proven that eliminating gluten from diet of people with autism greatly improves their health.

    iv.   Eliminates the chance of experiencing stomach pains for those who do not tolerate gluten intake.

    v.   It makes one conscious of the food him or her intakes and therefore gains a vast knowledge on nutrition. A person therefore tends to take food of higher energy.

Adopting a gluten free lifestyle is the best decision one can ever make. It shows that you care about your health as you will be taking healthy diets for each meal.

CHAPTER 6- BEST FOODS FOR THE GLUTEN FREE DIET

In this chapter we will endeavor to provide you with a variety and wholesome list of the best foods for living gluten free. Although it is sometimes difficult to ascertain which foods would be best if you are aware of the foods that can be included in the diet, it makes it a whole lot easier.

Grains & Flours

Arrowroot, amaranth, almond flour, brown rice, cassava, buckwheat, tef, bean flour, brown rice flour, chickpea flour, yucca, corn flour, cornmeal, cottonseed, tapioca flour, soy flour, rice and rice flour, pulses, sago, job's tears, flaxseed, Milo, quinoa, potato flour, millet and pea flour

Vegetables

Brussels sprouts, garlic, broccoli, cabbage, cauliflower, peas, lettuce, peppers, mushrooms, spinach, potato, sweet potatoes, pumpkin, radish, turnips, avocado, carrots, watercress, squash, artichokes, beans, asparagus, beets, onions, celery, okra, corn, parsley, eggplant and cucumber

Fruits

Mandarin, limes, oranges, mangoes, carobs, acai berries, cantaloupe, cherry, grapes, cranberries, kumquat, dates, kiwifruits, figs, quince, apples, strawberries, raspberries, tamarind, watermelon, apricot, tangerines, blueberries, lemons, bananas, papaya, persimmons, passion fruit, peach, pear, plums and pineapple

Poultry and Meat

Turkey, rabbit, quail, eggs, lamb, chicken, veal, goat, venison, duck, beef, buffalo, goose and pork

Dairy Foodstuffs

Plain yogurt, milk, butter is also gluten-free but make sure that you check on the gluten additives on the package, various types of cheese are gluten-free except for blue cheese

Food Additives

Gelatin, honey, algin, yeast, pectinase, soy lecithin, apple cider vinegar, guar gum, rosin, saffron, annatto, sucrose, xantham gum, karaya gum, maltodextrin, pectin, galactose, vanillin, lactose, acacia gum, tagatose, tragacanth gum, maltol, isinglass, lecithin, tara gum, ester gum, corn sweetener and white rice vinegar

Nutritional Supplements

Lipase, spirulina, papain, whey protein isolate, casein, hydrolyzed soy protein, hydrolyzed caseinate, casein, whey, pure vitamins, whey protein concentrate and soy protein isolate

Celiac disease is considered as a very common condition and a serious intestinal problem. Early diagnosis of the problem was difficult before but now a simple blood test can be done in order to detect the condition.

If someone in your family is suffering from the condition, visiting your physician for a checkup is necessary in order to conduct proper diagnosis. More importantly, follow a diet that contains the foods mentioned above in order to prevent the condition from worsening and to maintain a healthier body. You can also check the

Debbie Blaine

internet for various gluten-free recipes that you can opt for using the ingredients listed above, as part of your gluten-free diet.

CHAPTER 7- HOW TO REMAIN GLUTEN-FREE

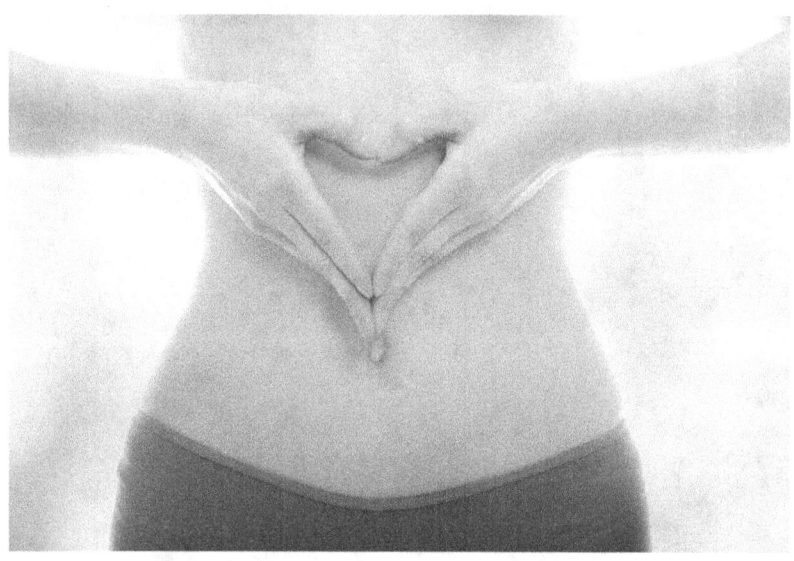

Allowed

Grains/Flours

Rice, corn (maize), soy, potato, tapioca, beans, garfava, sorghum, quinoa, millet, buckwheat, arrowroot, amaranth, teff, Montina®, flax, and nut flours

Oats

Research indicates that pure, uncontaminated oats consumed in moderation (up to 1/2 cup dry oats daily) are tolerated by most celiacs. Gluten-free oats are currently available in the United States. Consult your physician or dietician before including oats in your diet and for regular monitoring.

Distilled alcoholic beverages and vinegars are gluten-free. Distilled products do not contain any harmful gluten peptides. Research indicates that the gluten peptide is too large to carry over in the distillation process. This process leaves the resultant liquid gluten-free.

Wines and hard liquor/distilled beverages are gluten-free. Beers, ales, lagers and malt vinegars that are made from gluten-containing grains are not distilled and therefore, are not gluten-free. Gluten-free beers are available in the United States.

Not Allowed In Any Form

Wheat (einkorn, durum, faro, graham, kamut, semolina, spelt), rye, barley and triticale

Frequently overlooked foods that may contain gluten and need to be verified:

- Brown rice syrup
- Breading & coating mixes
- Croutons
- Energy Bars
- Flour or cereal products
- Imitation bacon
- Imitation seafood
- Marinades
- Panko (Japanese bread crumbs)
- Pastas
- Processed luncheon meats
- Sauces, gravies
- Self-basting poultry
- Soy sauce or soy sauce solids
- Soup bases
- Stuffings, dressing

- Thickeners (Roux)
- Communion wafers
- Herbal supplements
- Drugs & over-the-counter medications
- Nutritional supplements
- Vitamins & mineral supplements

If In Doubt Go Without!

When unable to verify ingredients or the ingredient list is unavailable - DO NOT EAT IT. Regardless of the amount eaten, it is not worth triggering your immune system and the damage to the small intestine that occurs every time gluten is consumed, whether symptoms are present or not. A person with celiac disease may have additional food sensitivity not related to gluten.

Many other products that you eat or that could come in contact with your mouth may contain gluten. These include:

- Food additives, such as malt flavoring, modified food starch, and others
- Lipstick and lip balms
- Medicines and vitamins that use gluten as a binding agent
- Postage stamps
- And Toothpaste

Whatever your reason for following a gluten-free diet, here are some tips that can help whether you are at home, at the store, or eating out:

At Home

Eat plenty of "plain" or unbreaded meat, fish, and poultry, as well as rice, fruits, and vegetables. These foods do not contain gluten.

Debbie Blaine

Consider using gluten-free versions of foods such as breads and pastas. You can find them at your local bakery or grocery store.

Check out gluten-free cookbooks. They can give you great ideas for adjusting recipes.

At the Store

Read the label before you purchase any food product. Some foods that might appear acceptable may contain gluten. A registered dietician can be a great resource for helping you learn how to read ingredient lists and can make suggestions about gluten-free alternatives.

If you still cannot tell by reading the label if a food contains gluten, check with the product's maker.

Some medicines contain gluten. Ask the pharmacist about whether or not the medicines you take contain wheat.

When Dining Out

Call the restaurant ahead of time and ask if it serves gluten-free foods.

Even if you call ahead, be sure to ask your server about whether the foods you order contain or are prepared with gluten.

Once you find a restaurant that meets your needs, stick with it. You'll become more familiar with the menu, and the wait staff can become more familiar with your dietary needs.

Keep in mind that following a gluten-free diet can seem overwhelming at first. You may have trouble figuring out what you can eat, what you need to avoid, and how to fit gluten-free foods into your diet. However, over time and with some patience and creativity, you will find that there are many foods that you can still enjoy.

Chapter 8- How to Shop

Finding out that one has Celiac disease does not have to be a limiting factor in one's life. All it takes is proper research and care in order to be able to shop for food and drinks that do not contain gluten and are safe for consumption.

Here are some shopping tips for living Gluten free:

Take the time to research as much as you can regarding Gluten rich foods - it would be best if you will have time to make informed decisions because this will directly affect your health. You need to take the time to know the foods that are rich in Gluten that you may avoid then. When shopping for food make sure that you will have ample time and that you are not rushing. In this way you would be able to read the labels. You need to set a time for shopping and go during off peak times so that it would be less stressful.

Create a list of brands that do not contain gluten and stick with it-you can research online regarding the foods that contain gluten. Not every product would be providing gluten-free labeling but it does not mean that they contain gluten which is why it would give you advantage to reach through the websites of this companies and research. If you are not sure of the product then it would be best to create a list of the phone number of the company and verify the ingredient. There is no need to worry because in an average supermarket you would be able to choose at least 2,000 products that are gluten free. You do not have to see Celiac disease as something that is restrictive you just have to be creative in finding out foods that can apply to your diet.

Spend more time in the produce section- it would be best if you can focus your energy on organic vegetables. Vegetables and fruits are packed with nutrients including fiber and folic acid and best of all they do not contain gluten.

Focus on getting items that did not go any processing- foods like dairy and eggs are naturally gluten free. But be careful in taking items that contain processed cheese, spreads as well as yogurt of those that contain labels like " enhanced milk" or those that contain thickeners or flavored egg substitutes.

Buy meats, poultry and fish- but before purchasing make sure that they do not contain any gluten-containing broths and flavoring. Avoid any imitation of crabmeat called the sirimi and avoid purchasing any marinated items.

Choose gluten free-grains- focus on getting gluten-free flours beans, pastas, quinoa, millet as well as teff. If you buy them in canned varieties make sure that they do not contain sauce.

If in case you plan to dine out you can research for restaurants that offer gluten free menus. There is a list of celiac friendly restaurants online. The menus are already posted online and you can even learn some tips on how these meals are created.

CHAPTER 9- THE GLUTEN FREE MEAL PLAN

To plan a meal, be it one meal or a series of meals that are gluten free, it is best to know what gluten is. Gluten is found in certain grains which people commonly eat, such as rye, wheat and barley. Manufacturers add gluten to foods low in protein and to sources and dressings to thicken them. The only option available to people who suffer from celiac and other gluten intolerances is to eat a gluten-free diet. What exactly does a gluten-free diet consist of? This article will attempt to create a typical menu for a gluten-free day.

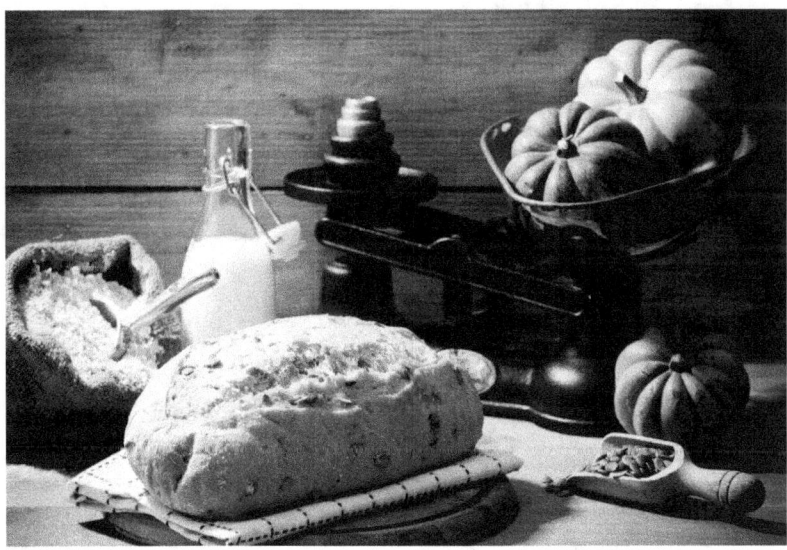

Gluten Free Foods

At the heart of a typical menu for gluten free day will be foods that are naturally gluten-free. These will typically be grains such as buckwheat, brown rice and others such as quinoa and amaranth. It is important that the list of foods include protein rich foods. Good gluten-free sources of protein include most nuts, meat milk, eggs, tofu and cheese. As always, vegetables and fruits must be part of any balanced diet. Corn and its products also are helpful if they are gluten-free.

Food for the Day

When planning a typical menu for a gluten free day, the best approach is to take the day as a whole. This makes it possible to include the needed daily intake of all the food groups (carbohydrates, fiber, proteins, and fats) and the essential vitamins, minerals, which the body needs. It also makes it possible to include the necessary amounts of sugar and fat that the body requires. The more balanced each of the meals is the healthier the overall daily nutrition will be.

Breakfast

Recent research has proved that a person's overall health when they start the day with a balanced breakfast. To make the most out of the available foods under a gluten-free diet, the idea of what foods people eat for breakfast, needs to change. For those who eat meat, sausages made from low-fat chicken, with some sautéed zucchini garnished with lemon juice would get the day off to a good start. For the vegetarians, a nice soup, preferably squash with some quinoa or other vegetable soup along with an egg and a slice of brown bread (toasted) would be just the right way to start the day.

Lunch

After the breakfast of chicken or egg and toast, the person has already consumed a healthy portion of protein. At lunch a robust salad with some low-fat cheese and some chicken preferably lean chicken for the health benefits. A small quantity of nuts or some avocado (a quarter should do) will add healthy fats. Dress the nuts and avocado with a mixture of raw apple cider vinegar a few herbs and half a teaspoon full of olive oil. Vegetarians who had the squash for breakfast would need a higher quantity of protein. For this 4 or 5 ounces chicken or a full portion of organic tofu is fine.

Dinner

For those who can get home in time, dinner provides the best time to experiment with the different recipes. Grilled fish (Salmon is a good choice) with lemon juice. Add salt and pepper to taste. Add a grilled vegetable skewer with some steamed gluten-free rice. These make for a nice way to end the day.

There it is a typical menu for a gluten-free day. With a little planning, the meals are both delicious and gluten-free.

CHAPTER 10- HOW GOING GLUTEN-FREE HELPS WITH WEIGHT LOSS

If you are a person who has unsuccessfully tried every single type of diet, ever invented, and failed miserably, you could read about the gluten free diet, which has been taking the world of weight loss by storm. This diet will allow you to eat everything that is wholesome, healthy and completely free of gluten. This kind of a diet was initially recommended for patients with an allergy towards gluten. When its weight loss benefits were discovered, the diet soon achieved a space in the weight loss category too.

What Are the Symptoms of a Gluten Allergy?

If you are planning to shift into a gluten free diet because you suspect that you have an allergy, then check the following symptoms before coming to your conclusion. The most common symptoms of a gluten allergy are gas formation bloating that gives you an uncomfortable feeling, an incessant feeling of tiredness and unexplainable weakness.

Though an allergy is one of the main reasons why people turn to a gluten free diet, some also choose it for its obvious health benefits.

"A gluten free diet is the best choice for losing weight along with improving your overall health".

What Can You Eat When On a Healthy Gluten Free Diet?

When on a gluten free diet, you should stick to wholesome, completely natural, unprocessed food items. This means that you will have to cut out most refined flours, especially the ones used in baked products.

Debbie Blaine

Here is a list of the gluten free and wholesome grains that you can add to your diet.

These will not add any extra calories but will make your diet more beneficial by including the ample amount of nutrients into it. Brown rice, Quinoa Wild rice, Amaranth, Millet, Teff, Corn and Buckwheat Oats

Choose Your Food Items with Care When On a Gluten Free Diet

Gluten free food items are expensive. Another factor that makes most of the people opt out of a gluten free diet is the addition of other materials into the gluten free food items. These additives can actually increase the amount of calories in the diet, making it more harmful than healthy. This is especially true if you are on a gluten free diet for weight loss purposes. The additives would completely destroy the purpose of being on this diet.

How Can I Be Sure That the Food Is Actually a Healthy Choice?

There are many certification programs that test the various products of the companies to ensure that they are gluten free and healthy.

What Are the Products That We Should Stay Away From?

When on a gluten free diet, try and stay away from bakery products, as they have to rely mostly on refined flours. There are many companies who add extra additives to make up for the absence of gluten products. These additives increase the calorie count and end up making the food items less healthy. You should opt for those manufacturers who use high fiber flours that are also more nutritious. These flours are usually made of beans, almonds, brown rice, amaranth, sorghum and quinoa.

Generally gluten free products are low on fiber, iron, vitamin D and B and calcium. The addition of the above mentioned healthy flours can make up for this nutritional deficiency.

Chapter 11- How to Start Living Gluten Free

You have probably heard about gluten free diet and you might be thinking that this is another passing diet fad. But in reality, living gluten free is more than just one of those diet trends that quickly emerge. Before going any further, let us have some of the basics about gluten.

What is Gluten?

Gluten is a type of protein which can be found in cereal grains like wheat, barley, rye and oats. It is the substance which is responsible for the dough's elastic texture as well as keeping sauces and soups thick in texture.

Why Excessive Gluten Intake May Be Bad

Since this protein composite, gluten, is quite sticky and has a glue-like nature, it can cause damage in the digestive system by inhibiting the body from taking in the vitamins and nutrients in the food we eat. The gluten attaches itself to the villi in the wall of the digestive tract thus making it difficult for the digestive system to do its job. As a result, your body may start to bloat and then you further weight gain may also be experienced.

Some Benefits of Living Gluten Free Today

Reduced Weight. Being gluten free has many benefits one of which is, reduced body weight. It can also decrease or totally diminished bloated bellies.

Provide Lasting Energy. Unlike foods with gluten, eating gluten free meals can provide you with lasting energy to help you go through the day. Meals with gluten actually slow us down rather than give us the energy we require.

How to Start Living Gluten Free Today

Carefully plan and research on the meals you eat. It is best to carefully assess all the foods you eat to separate the gluten rich from the gluten free foods. You should go with meals which include vegetables, meat and poultry, fish and fruits as well as dairy and eggs in limited quantities. There are also some other source of protein which are gluten free like tofu, beans and legumes and protein powders. Grains can still be taken but look for gluten free grain products and limit intake per day. Rice is a gluten free grain that you can also eat with meals.

There are some foods with gluten which we are hardly aware of. Avoid them. It is true. There are foods which actually have gluten in them; however, we are not aware of them. Some examples of the foods with hidden gluten in them are beer, croutons, soy sauce, and some dressings as well as marinades. You should always be keen in checking labels or researching about all the food you take.

Drink and party responsibly. No, this is not an advice for safe driving but actually for your gluten free living. As mentioned before beers are included on the list of foods with gluten so you must avoid beer at all cost. You can just go some wine or hard liquor if you need to drink. Drink moderately.

Once you have fully researched about the right food to include in your diet, build your daily meals. There are still a lot of foods which are gluten free which means that going on a gluten free diet will not bring you to starvation or force you to eat foods which you do not like. You will just start to eat healthier and stay gluten free and then reap its wonderful benefits. Start planning for the food you eat and start eating gluten free meals as early as possible.

It is not really that hard to start living a gluten free life. You will just need to be aware which the gluten rich foods are so you can avoid them completely and start building your gluten free meals. Start early to reap the wonderful benefits early.

Chapter 12- How to Deal with the Gluten-Free Child

Children are often the most difficult people to manage when it comes to maintaining a gluten free diet. This is because they like to go out with their friends, go to pizza parties, go to the movies, and all the while do not want to constantly worry about eating foods that may have gluten. When told they cannot have them at all, they feel completely isolated from their gluten eating friends.

So how can you keep kids happy around their friends, but still maintain a gluten free lifestyle?

The main key is to plan ahead. When your child is going to a birthday party, bring a few gluten free cupcakes so he or she can eat a sweet treat with the rest of the kids.

If going out to a pizza restaurant, call ahead and find out if they offer gluten free options, and order a special pizza just for your child. When the child goes to a friend's house for a sleepover, pack a backpack for him or her that is loaded with gluten free chips, gluten free cookies, gluten free brownies, and other fun snacks. This will allow for the full friend experience while still maintaining a safe and healthy lifestyle.

CONCLUSION

Hopefully this information has shown you how easy and how many health benefits there are to taking up a gluten free lifestyle. From lowering your risk for certain diseases, to having healthier children, and even having fewer digestive issues, there are a number of reasons to cut gluten from your diet.

Since more and more people are beginning to see the light and take part in this diet, the food choices have gotten more plentiful, restaurants have come on board, and meals are quite delicious.

In time you will realize this diet is quite simple and takes just a bit of extra planning, but the difference you will feel in your own body will astound you!

ABOUT THE AUTHOR

Debbie Blaine opted to live the gluten free lifestyle. She worked long hours as a trauma nurse and she simply found that the diet was more suited to her lifestyle. She knew persons who had no option but to live the gluten free lifestyle as they had celiac disease or gluten intolerance. This is what peaked her interest in what benefits this diet could have in the long run.

Her book outlines what she has discovered about the diet thus far and helps to reader to determine if the diet if really for them. It also educates the reader on what it means to HAVE TO live a gluten free lifestyle.

www.ingramcontent.com/pod-product-compliance
Lightning Source LLC
Chambersburg PA
CBHW071145280526
45787CB00003B/1408

* 9 7 8 1 6 3 2 8 7 4 5 9 7 *